HOW TO
CUT
KIDS' HAIR

How to ● Cut ● Kids' Hair ●

Nancy Hughes Clark

Illustrated by Celia Johnson

Addison-Wesley Publishing Company
Reading, Massachusetts • Menlo Park, California
London • Amsterdam • Don Mills, Ontario • Sydney

Library of Congress Cataloging in Publication Data

Clark, Nancy Hughes.
  How to cut kids' hair.

  1. Haircutting. I. Title.

TT970.C54 1984   646.7'242   83-25837
ISBN 0-201-10811-9

Designed by Larry Kazal K.C. Witherell, New York
Set in 10 point Times Roman by Wendy B. Wolf

ISBN 0-201-10811-9

ABCDEFGHIJ-AL-87654
First printing, February 1984

Contents

The day I paid $11 plus tip for my five-year-old's haircut — and realized that the three-year-old was also badly in need of a trim — was the day I started seriously to consider the possibility of learning how to cut my kids' hair. I'm sure that there are less expensive sources of haircuts than the comfortable-but-stylish East Side barber shop I was patronizing, but I also know there are *more* expensive options: the chic stylist from a fancy midtown salon who will pay a house call to your off-spring for a mere $100 an hour, for example. Depending on how much you're paying now, becoming your own barber can make a significant contribution to your family's balance of payments.

There are other incentives as well. Perhaps *your* children sit quietly and draw when forced to wait in a crowded shop, be it the barber shop or a shoe store, but mine don't. They make a beeline for the lollipop jar and then start investigating the equipment: items like plugged-in blow-dryers and sharp scissors. Waiting with small children is not my favorite pastime, and I reasoned that if I were doing the barbering, the frustration level would be considerably diminished.

A final reason for learning how to cut hair is psychological. There are certain stages of childhood when youngsters are naturally afraid of strangers, especially ones wearing official-looking smocks and wielding sharp instruments. Those are usually phases when parents simply throw up their hands and let their kids' hair grow (a perfectly reasonable decision when the alternative is a terrified child having a screaming tantrum). But as you develop hair-cutting expertise, you'll find that a trim can be a speedy, painless process, one that even a fearful child will endure if the trimmer is Mommy or Daddy.

Before picking up a pair of scissors, I

worried that it would be terribly difficult to learn the skill of cutting hair. After all, barbers and beauticians go to school and then apprentice before setting up a business. But I also realized that professionals have to be prepared to deal with an enormous variety of hair types, style preferences, and sophisticated "dos." As a family barber, you'll have considerably fewer "clients" to deal with, and chances are most of the hair types will be pretty similar. And you won't be trying any elaborate styles on your kids—the simpler the better, as you will see.

Like any precise craft, hair cutting does take practice to develop expertise, but depending on the number and enthusiasm of your family and friends, you probably have a willing pool of "heads" to experiment with, especially if you develop a liberal reward policy (see "Tricks of the Trade" in Chapter 2).

"The basic thing about cutting hair is to have the hand-tool co-ordination," explains Paul Maciag, co-owner of the chic Paul Molé barber shop on New York's Upper East Side and my expert consultant on the art of hair cutting. Paul's personal clientele includes both successful business and professional people and their children. "I feel I'm a pretty coordinated person," he continues, "but it still took a good deal of practice when I started out. I imposed a lot on friends!"

As you consider the haircut process, Paul reminds you that cuts ". . . are always symmetrical. What you do on the left, you do on the right. The sides and back should be pretty much the same, but the top can be longer or shorter, depending on your preference and the style you're cutting." He also has a warning: "The most difficult thing about cutting a child's hair is movement. If you don't really pay attention, you can poke him. You have to be ready to pull back your scissors at any second."

So a certain amount of dexterity is a prerequisite, caution is necessary, and so is a willingness to persevere. But acquiring the technique isn't hard, and the results can be enormously rewarding. You'll get the "feel" of hair cutting the very first time you try (I did), and after a few cuts, you'll begin to develop confidence. The finished product may look a little choppy at the beginning, but by your third or fourth attempt, no one will be able to tell that your child hasn't had an expensive cut at a fancy salon.

In the chapters that follow, you'll find

suggestions on how to choose the right style for your child's face, hair type, and personal preference; a rundown of the equipment you'll need (not much); the best location for trimming; general tips for shampooing, detangling, and combing; plus precise instructions on how to go about the cutting itself. And along the way, there are some "Tricks of the Trade" designed to calm, distract, or intrigue the squirmiest subject.

And then there are detailed directions for executing five different cuts, plus tips on trimming bangs and sideburns, creating braids and party styles, and dealing with hair-related disasters, major and minor.

Read through the book carefully; then turn to the style that seems most appropriate for your child and give it a try, following the instructions step by step.

1

Choose the Right Style

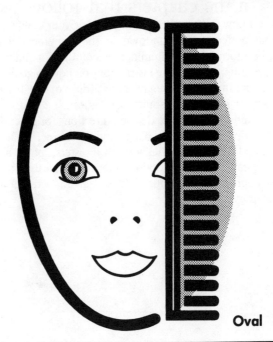

Oval

FACE SHAPES

Since the ideal of beauty is a perfect oval, one goal of any hairstyle is to make the wearer's face *appear* oval, whatever its actual shape. To perform a quick check of your child's facial structure, hold a comb vertically along one side. If her face is pear-shaped, heart-shaped, or diamond-shaped, there will be an area of chin and/or forehead which the comb doesn't touch. That's the area that needs to be filled in by a hairstyle to create the illusion of an oval.

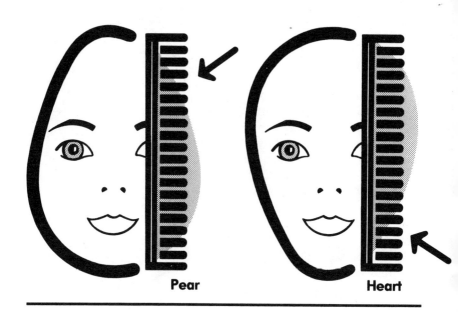

Pear

Heart

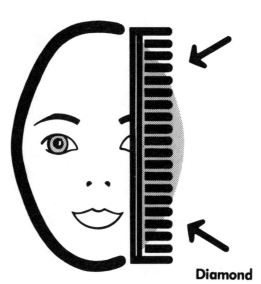

Diamond

CHOOSE THE RIGHT STYLE

A **pear-shaped face** needs some volume of hair at the brow to balance and camouflage the square, determined jaw below. Good styles for a pear-shaped face include the One-Length Cut (Chapter 4), parted and brushed away from the face (shown at right); the Short Blunt Cut (Chapter 5), done very short (shown below); and the Blunt Cut (Chapter 6), worn straight with full bangs (shown lower right).

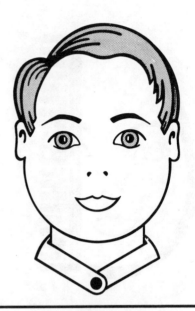

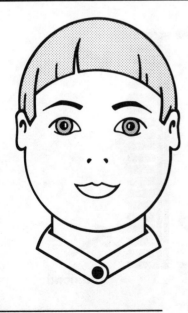

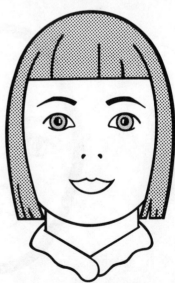

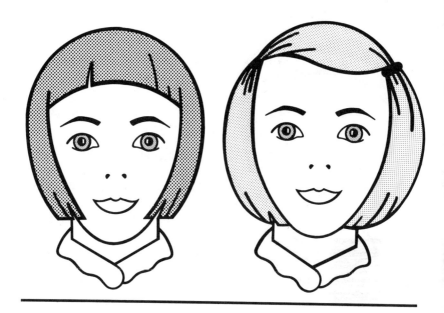

A **heart-shaped face**, on the other hand, looks best with some fullness at the chin. Good styles for the heart-shaped face include the Short Blunt Cut done chin-length (shown above); the Blunt Cut parted, with fullness at the chin (shown above right); and for wavy hair, a medium-length Layered Cut (Chapter 7), also with fullness at the chin (shown at right).

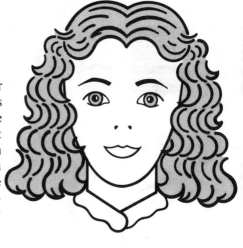

CHOOSE THE RIGHT STYLE

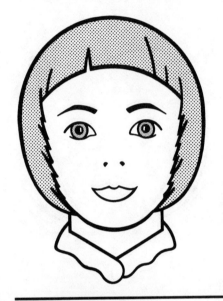

A **diamond-shaped face** requires "filling in" both top and bottom. Good styles for a diamond-shaped face include the Short Blunt Cut done medium (shown at left); the Blunt Cut with bangs and fullness at the chin (shown lower left); and the Layered Cut with extra volume at the chin (shown below).

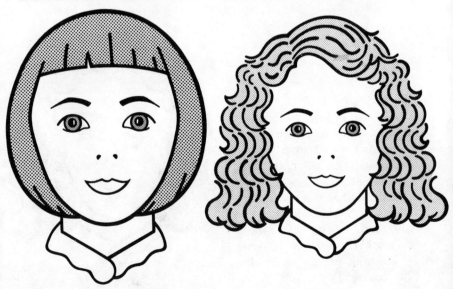

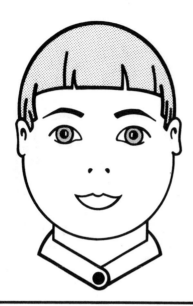

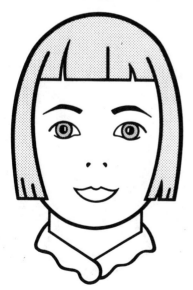

Many children have either a **round** or **squarish facial structure,** and covering the hairlines at the top and on the sides helps to camouflage the fullness. Bangs cut narrow, just to the outer edges of the eyes, have a slenderizing effect.

CHOOSE THE RIGHT STYLE

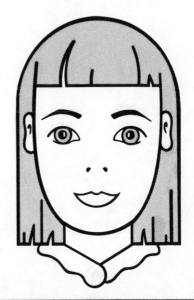

A **rectangular face** needs fullness at
the sides and back, and bangs can
help to minimize the length. Bangs
cut wide, past the temples, add
width to a slender face.

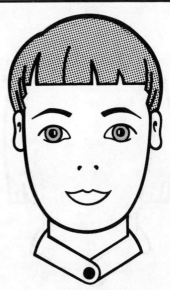

Also remember that creating an oval illusion is a three-dimensional goal. Your child's head should look well-proportioned from all four sides, not just from the front. If your little girl has long hair and a predilection for pony tails, for instance, consider her profile as you perform the task: the pony tail should be positioned to balance her features and complement the overall shape of her head.

Study your subject from all angles before deciding on the style to try. If you're torn between two possibilities, one shorter than the other, attempt the longer cut first. That way you have a fallback position.

HAIR TYPES AND TEXTURES

The crowning glory or, more likely, hopeless mop that is your child's head of hair may be dry, normal, or oily — those are the three generally recognized hair *types*. The self-evident rule governing the care and cleaning of hair is that if it's oily, you wash it more often. As those of us with small children know, however, it is possible to tolerate a greater accumulation of dirt, grease, or even gum and peanut butter in a youngster's hair than in one's own, especially if the youngster in question treats shampoo time as a kind of torture unequaled since medieval days. Fortunately, it is the onset of adolescence that usually sets the oil glands to working overtime, so few little kids have really oily hair.

In addition to *type*, there are five hair *textures*, which do occur in all ages in various combinations: fine and coarse, straight, wavy, and curly. To a certain extent, your child's hair type and texture may determine the most appropriate style for him.

Very fine, thin hair usually looks best in a relatively short cut. The shortness gives it more volume, and it appears thicker.

Coarse hair may be worn long or short, but it generally looks best in a simple, geometric cut rather than in layers. The weight of the hair flattens out the layers and the results look choppy.

Very curly hair, on the other hand, needs some layering for control — cut all one length, it tends to bush out wildly. If you have a little girl with lots of curly hair, you might consider as short a cut as you can get away with. Long, curly hair attracts tangles that can be literally impossible to comb through.

Wavy and **straight** hair are the most adaptable; almost any style is suitable.

CHOOSE THE RIGHT STYLE

The most important element of a child's hairdo, however, is ease of maintenance. "Children's hair should be maintenance-free," says expert Paul Maciag. "After all, it's tough enough for *adults* to maintain elaborate styles, much less children." So the watchword is simplicity. All of the cuts in this book are wash-and-wear styles — none requires any fancy blow-drying or setting. Most can be done at different lengths. A blunt cut, for instance, could be done on chin-length hair or on shoulder-length hair with equally appealing results. The one-length cut can be done short on very curly hair to produce an Afro, or slightly longer on straight hair with results that are distinctly preppy.

PERSONAL PREFERENCE

Not just hair type but body type, too, should be taken into account when choosing a style for your son or daughter. Very short hair on pudgy or solid people, kids included, makes them look bottom-heavy. And the same short hair on an extremely thin youngster makes him seem to vanish into thin air. For both body types, a softer, medium-length style would be the most flattering.

Personal preference is another factor to consider, especially for little girls. If your daughter is a tomboy — the star pitcher on the local Little League team, for instance — urge her to consider a style that is either quite short or quite long, rather than anything in between. The short style is, by definition, manageable, and shoulder-length hair can always be braided or secured in a pony tail during athletic endeavors or strenuous play.

If, on the other hand, she's ultrafeminine, she'll probably want at least chin-length hair and probably more of a mane so that she can spend long hours monopolizing the bathroom while she curls and fusses and experiments.

A child who is disaster-prone presents another set of problems. If she can't get through a week without someone's Tootsie Roll Pop landing in her hair and if she seems to have discovered the mud pack as a routine scalp treatment, the only sane course is a really short cut.

The same holds true for children who actively detest shampoos or baths (or both). Short hair may well get just as dirty as long hair, but somehow it doesn't get nearly so unsavory-looking.

If short hair is in your long-tressed girl's future, one suggestion: reduce it gradually, over the course of three or four haircuts. To be radically shorn all at once is a real trauma and shouldn't be inflicted on anyone who has even the slightest qualms. From a practical point of view, such a maneuver could set the cause of your at-home hair-cutting project back several months. So proceed with restraint, even if there *is* bubble gum right up near her bangs. (There are tips on how to get rid of it in Chapter 9.)

I haven't been concentrating on little boys because, generally speaking, you have less leeway with a male child than you do with a girl. The days when you could get away with shoulder-length curls on Junior until age eight are long past, and there aren't a whole lot of variations in boys' haircuts. It's either straight, wavy, or curly, but it's usually pretty short. The negative side of that coin is that you can't use your little boy's hairstyle to balance his face shape or his features except by choosing to comb the bangs down or to the side (a very important choice, I hasten to add — as we've seen, bangs can make an enormous difference in appearance). On the positive side, you have all the practical advantages of a trim, manageable style.

Short haircuts on kids have a lot going for them. In fact, the only drawback I can think of is the need for frequent cuts. But since *you're* doing the cutting, that's not even a liability. It's just a chance for you to perfect your skills!

2

The At-Home Barber Shop

NECESSARY EQUIPMENT

No major capital expenditure is required to start cutting your family's hair, but you do need a few items, which you may already have.

A dime-store **barber's cape**, probably made of plastic with ties at the neck, is a good and inexpensive investment. A towel, fastened securely around your child's neck with a safety pin, is an adequate substitute, but you'll find that the cut hair clings to it doggedly, no matter how vigorously you shake it after the fact, and as a result, you wind up with another towel to launder every time you give a haircut. The barber's cape, on the other hand, sheds hair like a duck's back sheds water, and all it ever needs is an occasional wipe, especially if your children like to eat popsicles while being trimmed. In addition, you can manage a tighter seal around the neck with a garment designed for that purpose and thus avoid the squirming and complaining that are unavoidable results of tiny hairs stuck to a child's neck and shoulders.

A **spray bottle** is another necessity. Children's hair dries incredibly fast, and, at least at the beginning, you'll be cutting at a less-than-breakneck pace. So you'll need to keep your subject's hair wet as you go along. (I'll explain

Tricks of the Trade

If you have more than one child, collect as many spray bottles as you have kids. They become treasured items (the source of incredible battles if there aren't enough), and they're wonderful playthings at bath time and outside in the summer. (But at no other times or places, if you value your furniture finish, your upholstery, etc.) You might also personalize each one with a youngster's name and have terrific, decorative substitutes for water pistols.

why in a minute.) If you want to, you can buy a bottle designed for misting plants, or use the one you already have, if you're a plant person. Or you can remember to save the bottle next time you finish your supply of Windex, Fantastik, or whatever. Naturally, you will rinse out a detergent bottle very carefully, but once it's clean, it will serve the purpose perfectly.

For children with medium to long hair, you'll need some **hair clips** or **coated rubber bands** or both to help you with the sectioning process. Clips are probably more practical for fine hair, rubber bands for thick or coarse hair.

A good **comb** is a must. "But I have a million combs around the house," you say. True, but you may not have one that is about eight inches long and

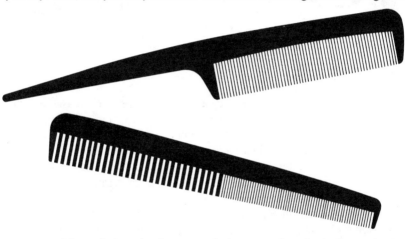

narrow, with gradations in the spaces between teeth: a barber's comb. As one who has tried with a plain old pocket comb, I can testify that it's easier to control the section you're cutting with the kind of comb illustrated above.

Some barbers and stylists prefer what's called a "rattail" comb, and you may, too. The tail can be used to part and create sections, so what you lose in not having the teeth gradations may be compensated for by the maneuverability. You'll probably want to experiment with a couple of different styles and pick the one that feels most comfortable. After all, how much can a couple of combs cost?

Suggests expert Paul Maciag, "I would recommend that people use a larger comb rather than a smaller one, since most children's hair is on the

THE AT-HOME BARBER SHOP

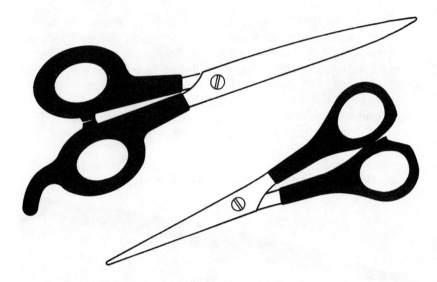

long side. With a longer comb, you can pick up more and it's easier to work with. Then when you get to the nape of the neck, switch to a narrower one."

Scissors are, of course, the most crucial item, and the one that can cost the most. You need sharp, high-quality barber shears in order to make a success of your hair-cutting project. The old shears in the kitchen drawer that you use for trimming flowers and opening flour bags simply will not do.

Barber shears are narrow, sharply pointed scissors about seven inches long, usually with a curved finger rest on the finger loop. Good scissors are a precision tool, and precise alignment of the two blades is necessary for them to work properly. When you try out a pair of scissors, make sure they open and shut easily—the tension shouldn't be too tight or too loose—for finger-tip control. They should be lightweight and feel comfortable in your hand: the thumb and finger loops should fit *your* thumb and finger. They should open and close smoothly, with the same amount of pressure from the pivot to the tip and back. Check the finish—there should be no rough spots or protruding screws or rivets.

Left-handed would-be barbers have a special problem. Though many scissors these days are labeled "right- or left-handed," I'm told it just isn't so. If ordinary scissors aren't comfortable in your left hand, seek out a special left-handed store that can supply tools that really fit.

THE AT-HOME BARBER SHOP

A smaller version of barber shears are called "styling scissors," and they look very much the same, but without the finger rest (see illustration). I strongly recommend investing in a pair of each, since the smaller scissors are much easier to use when you're trimming around the neck and sideburns, or cutting bangs. But you need the larger shears to make the quick inch-or-longer cuts over the rest of the head — to attempt a whole haircut with styling scissors would be to invite finger fatigue and a very cranky, bored child.

As to brands of scissors, *Consumer Reports* (July 1983) recommended barber shears by Singer (about $14), by Marks (about $18), and by Hoffritz (about $20). The magazine also suggested having scissors professionally sharpened when necessary, or, if that's too expensive a proposition, simply buying a new pair when the old one gets dull.

SETTING UP SHOP

Plan to do your hair cutting somewhere with plenty of light and with relatively few encumbrances — you need to be able to move all around a seated child, without bumping your elbows on bookshelves, chandeliers, hot saucepans, or assorted siblings.

Tricks of the Trade

If you're especially flexible yourself and have a healthy back, consider cutting your youngster's hair in the bathtub. After the shampoo, empty the water, dry the child off, put some nylon net over the drain to catch stray hairs, and put in a stool or something for the child to sit on. After the cut is complete, you can simply rinse off the now-clipped kid, gather up the hair in the nylon, and toss it away. With nude barbering, you don't even need a cape around the neck!

Be sure that the spot you decide on has a bare floor — wood, linoleum, ceramic tile, or the like. *Never* cut on a carpeted surface — you'll be vacuuming up hairs forever. And even on a sleek surface, spread out a generous layer of newspaper. It's *so* much easier to wad up the debris and throw it away than to look for the dustpan, get out a broom, and sweep.

THE AT-HOME BARBER SHOP

Position the child on a stool, a booster chair, or a phone book—his or her head should be high enough so that you can reach it comfortably, without stooping, bending, or contorting yourself.

To clean up afterward, most professionals have a whisk broom of some sort to brush off those hairs that seem to have lodged permanently on your offspring's neck. A brisk rub or two with a towel is somewhat effective, or you might try removing the offending hair with the hose of your vacuum cleaner, if the idea doesn't terrify your little one. Blow-dryers do the job, too.

Tricks of the Trade

If you haven't yet thrown it away, try using the high chair as your barber stool, at least for kids up to about five or so (beyond that age, it might be quite a squeeze). The chair positions the child at just the right height, and the tray provides a surface onto which you can put something interesting—a puzzle, perhaps—for distraction. Even more important, the tray immobilizes the child considerably, minimizing twists and squirms.

PREPARATION

There are two very good reasons for cutting hair while it's wet. First, wet hair sticks together, and when you snip a bit off, it won't fly all over the place, it will drop neatly onto the cape or the floor or wherever. Second, since it does shrink in volume and stick together when wet, it's far easier to see the line you're cutting and keep it straight or curved.

Therefore, the first step in a good haircut is a good shampoo. Wash your child's head thoroughly, paying special attention to the scalp. Get everything clean. (I stress this only because I've been horrified to discover cradle cap on a three-year-old—my own—and it's not a pretty sight!)

If a shampoo is, itself, a trauma in your household, consider separating that operation from the haircut. Hair doesn't have to be clean to be cut, after all. It just has to be wet. And you can do that with a spray bottle.

Wet hair, especially on a youngster, is often tangled hair, and the spray-on or comb-through cream rinses are heartily recommended. Few things are more unpleasant than combing through wet tangles, so use whatever you can find at the local drugstore to make the task easier.

**Tricks
of the
Trade**

Since shampoo time can be problematic, here are some consumer-tested hints for minimizing the wear and tear—if not on you, at least on *them*:

- Use a well-cleaned syrup or dishwashing-detergent bottle with a pull-up top for your shampoo. It gives you one-hand control as you open and close it.

- Especially in winter, float the (closed) shampoo bottle in the bathtub for a few minutes before using it. The shampoo itself won't be such a cold shock to a young scalp.

- Apply the shampoo with a sponge so it doesn't get in your child's eyes as it's going on.

- To rinse, try a child's watering can. (Assuming your child is willing to tip his head back. The whole point, after all, is to keep the water out of his eyes, right? At least that's the objection I've always had to cope with.)

- Another possibility is to put just a couple of inches of water in the tub in the first place so that your child can lie flat on his back for the rinsing process and still be well out of the water.

- An empty plastic gallon milk jug, filled with water and sunk to the bottom of the tub, can serve as a headrest come rinsing time, and some children are perfectly happy to have water in their faces while wearing swimming goggles. For others, a washcloth held tightly over the eyes does the trick.

- If your youngster is really and truly terrified of the whole procedure, try wrapping him in a huge, fluffy beach towel and positioning him flat on the kitchen counter next to the sink (face up, naturally). The towel will give him some comfort and security, and you can rinse his hair off with the sink spray.

The best technique for combing just-washed hair is to use as wide-toothed a comb as you have; then start at the bottom of the hair and work up gradually toward the scalp to avoid both breakage of the hair, and wear and tear on your nerves. (This is the moment when you'll really be tempted to try something *very* short on natural curls.)

ATMOSPHERE

The at-home haircut should be a pleasant shared experience, not a trial, and a relaxed attitude is important. *Never* experiment when you're tense or anxious or angry—that's courting disaster. And don't force it. If the time isn't right, wait for another time.

Don't underestimate the value of distractions. Play music or put on a storytelling record. Wait for a favorite program and turn on the television. Set up a large mirror so your child can see himself and everything that's happening, if that's a better way to approach it.

Try putting a Halloween mask on your youngster and then seating him in front of a mirror. The mask itself provides distraction and also keeps stray hairs out of his face and cold scissors away from his skin. Since you know your child, you can guess what project or activity may work to keep him calm and diverted.

Paul Maciag suggests that the first time you try your hand at barbering, make it a joint effort and a very brief one, at that. He recommends that one parent stand by with a gentle hand on the child's jaw, while the other

Tricks of the Trade

Institute a liberal rewards policy. It's not for nothing that barber shops catering to children have jars full of lollipops and other goodies. I find it effective to space the treats: "One pretzel now, before we begin, and then two cookies in the middle—and some juice, if you're thirsty—and a piece of candy when we're all done. If you've been a very good boy." There are certain times during childhood, I believe, when blatant bribery is the only approach to take. Crowded supermarkets qualify, and so do those beginning haircuts!

dampens the bangs, combs them straight down, and trims. This procedure gives everyone a feeling for the process, but doesn't require too much time or concentration during the initial attempt.

Another technique for trimming bangs is to use not-too-sticky "hairdo" tape. (It's available in all drugstores.) Tape low across the bangs and cut neatly above the tape. If objections are raised to that because the child can feel the scissors against his skin, try placing a thin piece of cardboard between forehead and hair so that the cold metal doesn't offend.

A psychological recommendation is to call the process a "trim" rather than a "cut"; sometimes small children make negative associations with the word "cut" and worry that they will be hurt.

CUTTING TECHNIQUE

There are a few basic cutting techniques that you need to learn, basics that are used for all the different haircuts in this book. First, stand behind your seated child and comb his wet hair straight back. With the comb in your right hand (reverse this procedure if you are left-handed), take a small section of hair—say an inch wide and an inch deep—from the center front of the forehead. (This is the starting point for most of the styles described

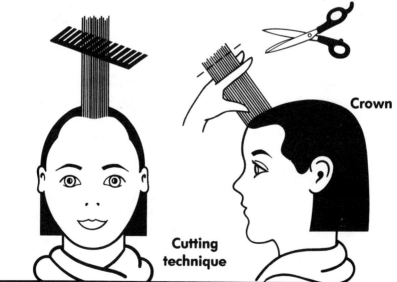

Crown

Cutting technique

later. There will be detailed instructions for any variations.) Once that section is neatly combed up, hold it between the fore- and third finger of your left hand. Your fingers should be pointing in the direction of a center part — toward the crown — and should be parallel to the top of the head.

Put the comb down in an easily accessible place. Pick up the scissors with your right (comb) hand and snip neatly and quickly across the section between your fingers, parallel to the head.

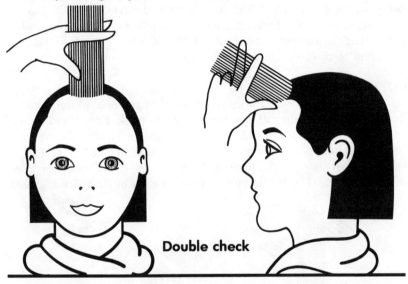

Double check

To check your cut and make sure it is even, comb the cut section up again, this time holding it with your fingers crosswise above the forehead, still parallel to the top of the head. The cut edge should still be straight and even. Every cut you make can be checked in this fashion to ensure precision — just switch your fingers from front-to-back position to side-to-side position.

Always cut hair above or in front of your fingers so that the cut hair falls away from you and down. Never cut behind your fingers or between fingers and scalp. And always cut with the same hand that holds the comb. At the beginning, this technique will require putting down and picking up the comb and the scissors over and over, but as you become skilled, you may be able to handle both at once.

THE AT-HOME BARBER SHOP

I recommend cutting quite small sections, but never more hair than an inch-by-inch square. The smaller the cuts you make, the more precise will be the results. If you cut a large hunk, the line will be noticeable in the finished hairdo, but if you're snipping small pieces, all the cuts will blend together for a polished, finished style.

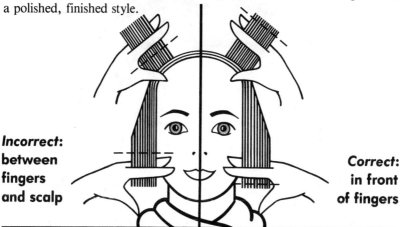

Incorrect: **between fingers and scalp**

Correct: **in front of fingers**

While trimming around ears or on bangs, place the back of your left hand against the child's head and cut over the palm of that free hand so that the scissors don't touch the child's skin. (Or use the cardboard technique.)

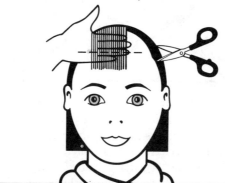

A final suggestion: Practice using two fingers instead of scissors before you make your first cut. The risk-free trial run will help you get the feel of hair cutting and develop confidence.

3

The One-Cut Cut

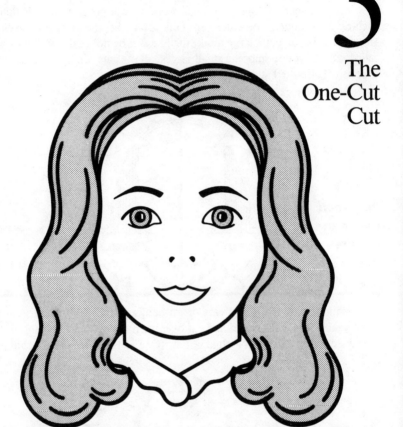

An extremely easy cut to do, this style works only for be-low-shoulder-length hair that is slightly wavy. The result is a tousled, semi-layered look, and natural curl will compensate for any minor imperfections in the line.

This is an ideal "beginning" haircut to try, especially if your subject is a rambunctious little girl who has a hard time sitting still for more than a minute and a half. Once you've developed confidence and expertise, you might want to try a long Layered Cut instead.

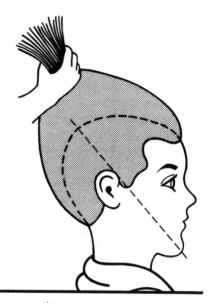

1 Comb the wet hair straight up, grasping all of it with your left hand (assuming you're right-handed) slightly in front of the crown. (The crown is the top of your head, the point a straight line drawn starting at the chin and passing through the ear would touch. Let's call that line the "crown line.") Keep even tension on the hair with your non-cutting hand.

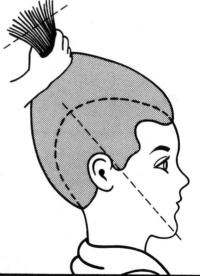

2 Cut all the hair straight across, parallel to the top of the head, above your hand.

3 Let the hair fall naturally. The front hair will, naturally, be shorter than the back hair: the effect is layered and casual.

4

The One-Length Cut

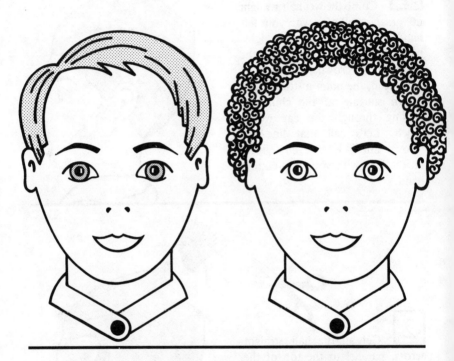

This cut is a very basic one, suitable for short to medium hair of all types and textures. It involves cutting all the hairs on your child's head approximately the same length. If the hair in question is straight or wavy, the result will be a neat, Ivy League style, either with or without bangs, depending on how you comb it. If your child has extremely curly hair, the same cut will result in an "Afro" style, either conservative or full-blown, depending on the length you choose.

THE ONE-LENGTH CUT

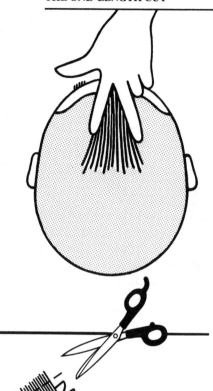

1 Starting at the center front, comb up a section of hair that is about an inch wide and an inch or less deep. Hold the section betwcen the fore- and third finger of your non-cutting hand, fingers pointing toward the crown.

2 Cut the section straight across, whatever length you have chosen.

THE ONE-LENGTH CUT

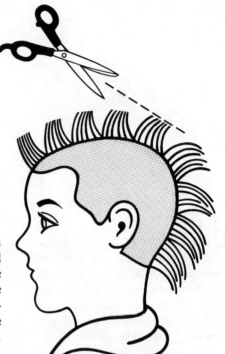

3 Comb up another section of the same size, directly behind the first and including a few of the already-cut hairs. Cut it the same length as the first. Continue, section by section, back over the crown and to the nape of the neck.

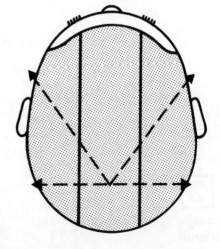

4 Return to the front of the head and part one side in triangular sections, radiating from the crown like the spokes of a wheel.

5   Starting at the crown, comb a small section of hair in the frontmost triangle, including a few of the cut hairs from the center section. Cut it the same length, following the contour of the head.

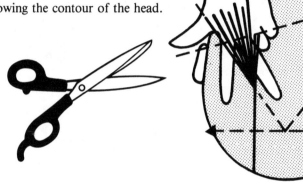

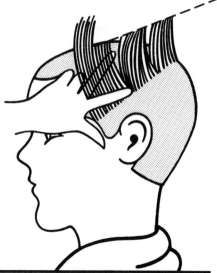

6   Continue in that section, inch by inch, cutting forward to the hairline.

THE ONE-LENGTH CUT

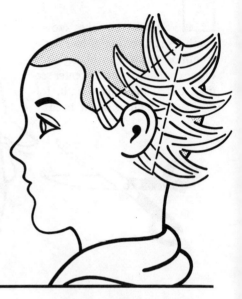

7 Cut the next section in the same fashion, then the backmost section, always keeping the holding fingers pointed toward the crown, the cuts all parallel to the head.

8 Repeat the whole process on the other side.

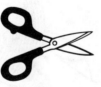

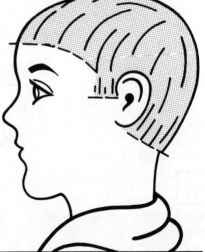

9 With styling scissors, trim the nape of the neck, the sideburns and around the ears (on boys), and the bangs. If the hair is very curly, you may want to check the outline and do some fine trimming once it's dry.

5

The Short Blunt Cut

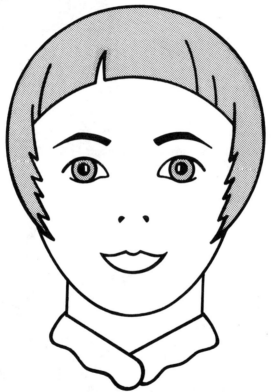

This style works extremely well on coarse or straight hair—short or medium length. It's a blunt cut that looks as good on little boys as on girls. Since the bangs are an integral part of the cut, don't choose this style if your child can't stand hair on his or her face.

THE SHORT BLUNT CUT

1 To accomplish the sectioning required for this cut, envision your child's head as a wagon wheel, with the center at the point of the crown. The sections will radiate out like spokes of the wheel.

2 Starting at the crown, section the hair into three concentric circles, each comprising about a third of your child's hair. Secure the crown section with a clip or covered rubber band; then proceed to the middle circle and divide it into four or five equal sections, securing each one with a clip or band. Comb the final circle down around the face.

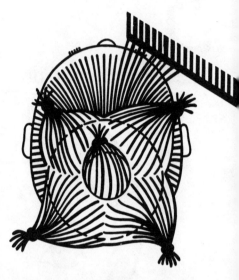

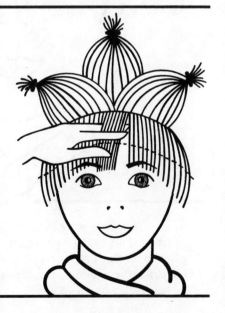

3 Decide on the length you want and make your first cut in the center of the forehead. Continue around, keeping tension on the hair with your holding fingers. Including a small part of the previous section in each section, you cut so that you have a length guide for every cut. Trim around the ears (unless the length you've chosen covers the ears).

THE SHORT BLUNT CUT

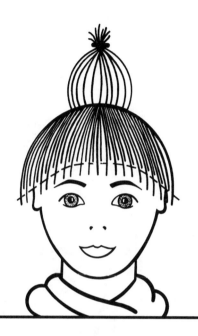

4 Once the first section is cut evenly all around the head, remove the clips or bands from the center circle and comb that hair down over the now-cut layer. Starting at the center front, cut this layer in the same fashion as the first, but make it slightly longer — about a quarter of an inch. Judge length by comparing with the already-cut hair underneath.

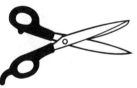

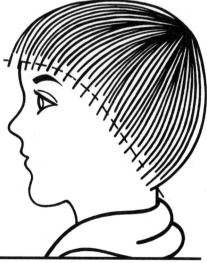

5 Now release the final, topmost section, comb it down, and cut evenly around, starting at the center front, as you did with the other two circles. Again, make this layer of hair about a quarter of an inch longer than the middle layer.

6
The Blunt Cut

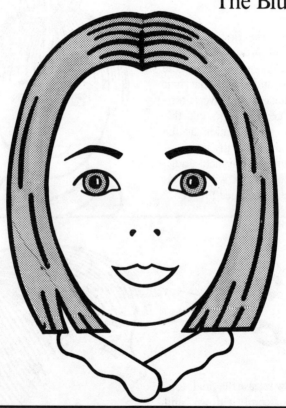

This is *the* cut for girls with straight hair, medium to long. It's easy to do and can be worn with or without bangs. (For how to incorporate bangs, see Chapter 8. Here, the assumption is a hair-off-the-face look, which can be dressed up with barrettes, hair bands, ribbons, and the like.)

THE BLUNT CUT

1. Comb the hair straight back; then make a horizontal part all the way around the head, starting at the middle of the ear. Comb the top section up and secure it with a clip or band. Comb the bottom section down.

2. Beginning at one side, take a small section of hair—no more than an inch—between your fingers, keep some tension on the hair, and cut it evenly straight across, just below your fingers.

3   Repeat with the adjacent hair, including a few of the already-cut hairs in the new section to keep the length uniform.

4   Cut all the way around the head, either keeping the line perfectly straight or incorporating a slight curve toward the center of the back. (A blunt cut may be precisely even all around or it may be slightly longer in the front or slightly longer in the back. Decide which style will best complement the shape of your child's head and face.)

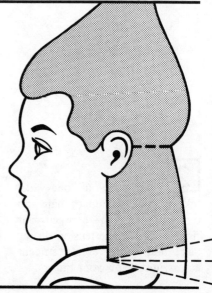

THE BLUNT CUT

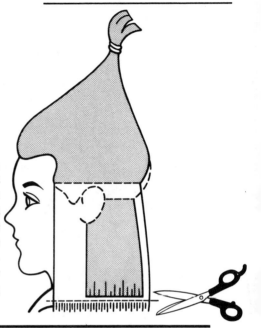

5 Release the top section, but keep control of it, and make a new section about a half-inch above the first—that is, about a half-inch above the ear. Secure the remaining top section and comb the new layer straight down. Starting at one side, cut this layer exactly as the first, but make it about a quarter of an inch longer.

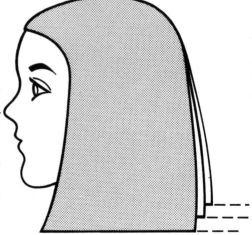

6 Continue bringing down half-inch sections and cutting them evenly around the head until all of the hair has been cut. (You will need to make a center part when you reach the last layer.) Make each succeeding layer a quarter-inch longer than the one before to achieve a slightly turned-under look.

THE LAYERED CUT

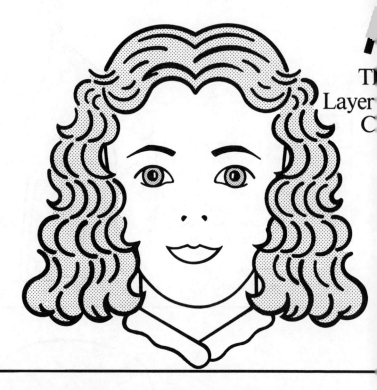

TI
Layer
C

A layered cut is versatile, practical, and looks good on a wide assortment of youngsters. Its main advantage from the parent's point of view is that although it looks relatively long, it's actually quite short, and therefore manageable. So for a child who's disaster-prone or shampoo-shy, but who resists really short hair, the layered cut may be the answer.

It's a good style for thick, wavy hair, and also good for thin hair since the layers add volume and fullness. It can provide considerable control for curly hair, but it's not so successful for either stick-straight or really kinky tresses.

The Layered Cut is slightly more difficult to execute than the preceding styles, but once you've gained some experience and confidence, you won't find it too hard.

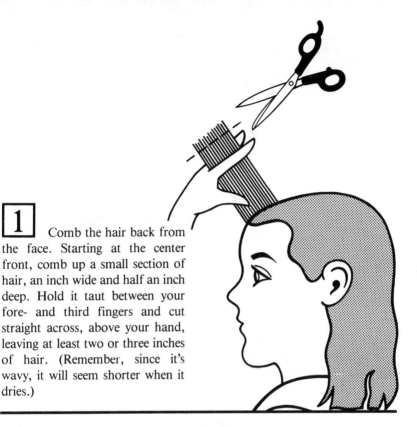

1 Comb the hair back from the face. Starting at the center front, comb up a small section of hair, an inch wide and half an inch deep. Hold it taut between your fore- and third fingers and cut straight across, above your hand, leaving at least two or three inches of hair. (Remember, since it's wavy, it will seem shorter when it dries.)

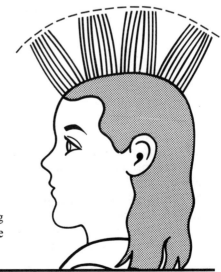

2 Continue back, cutting section after section the same length until you reach the crown.

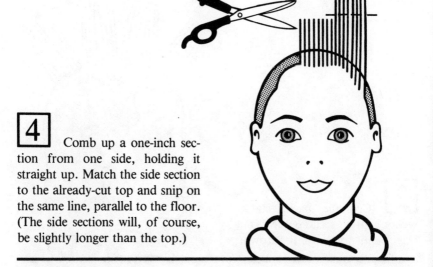

3 Go back to the front and make a side-to-side part running from ear to ear. Comb the hair in front of the ears forward.

4 Comb up a one-inch section from one side, holding it straight up. Match the side section to the already-cut top and snip on the same line, parallel to the floor. (The side sections will, of course, be slightly longer than the top.)

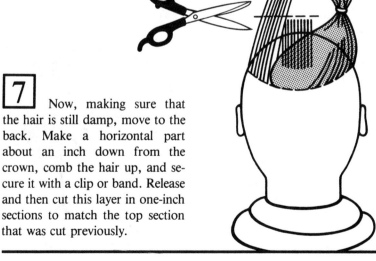

5 Comb up another one-inch section from the side. Cut along the same line as the previous cut. Repeat with any remaining side hair.

6 Repeat the process on the other side.

7 Now, making sure that the hair is still damp, move to the back. Make a horizontal part about an inch down from the crown, comb the hair up, and secure it with a clip or band. Release and then cut this layer in one-inch sections to match the top section that was cut previously.

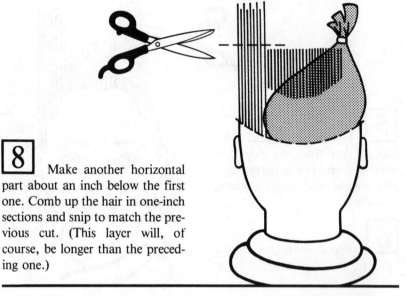

8 Make another horizontal part about an inch below the first one. Comb up the hair in one-inch sections and snip to match the previous cut. (This layer will, of course, be longer than the preceding one.)

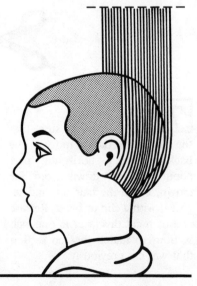

9 Keep repeating the process inch by inch until all the back layers are cut. Each cut should be made above the crown, parallel to the floor.

THE LAYERED CUT

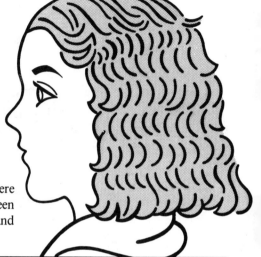

10 Check to make sure there is no awkward transition between the shorter layers of the front and the longer layers of the back.

8

Bangs and Sideburns

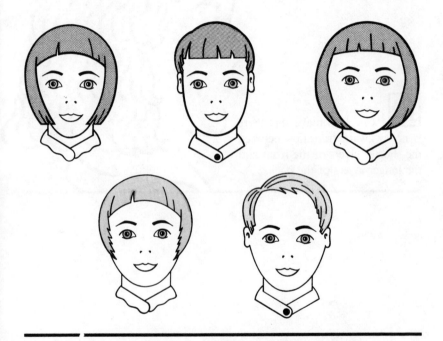

Many of the haircuts just described have their own built-in bangs, and sideburns are taken care of by the instructions to trim around the ears. (Since little boys don't develop actual sideburns until puberty, when facial hair starts to appear, they are an illusion that you, as the barber, must create.) But if you have a little girl with a Blunt Cut, or a One-Cut Cut, and if the sideburns that result from your "trimming" aren't precise enough for you, here are some additional pointers.

Bangs

1

Starting at the crown, part the front hair in a triangular section and comb it forward. (The triangle can be as wide at the front as you wish — to add width to a slender face; or as narrow — to minimize a round face.)

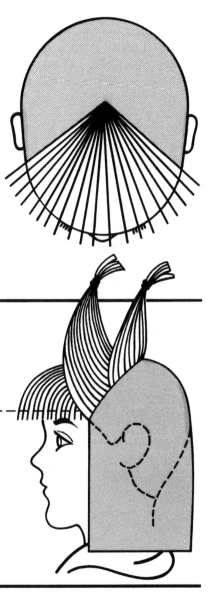

2

Divide the triangular section into three layers, securing the back two with clips or bands. Comb the front layer down over the face and decide how long you want the bangs. Cut carefully across, keeping your hand between the scissors and your child's forehead to prevent poking.

BANGS AND SIDEBURNS

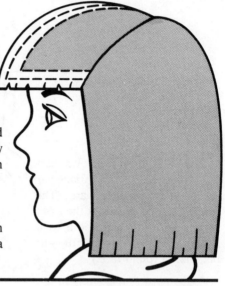

3   Release the next layer and comb it down, then cut it carefully and evenly a quarter of an inch longer than the hair underneath.

4   Repeat the process with the third layer, again making it a quarter-inch longer.

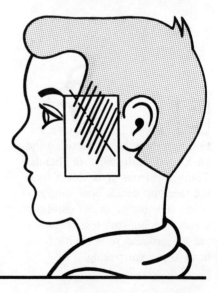

Sideburns

1   Holding a small piece of cardboard in your left hand (a three-by-five card will do nicely), comb the hair that will become the sideburn forward over the cardboard. Cut neatly from bottom to top.

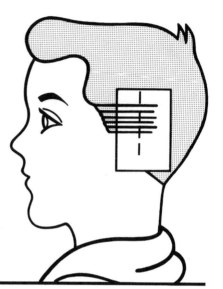

2 Now comb the hair back toward the ear, placing the cardboard between hair and ear to prevent poking. Trim again.

9

Finishing Touches

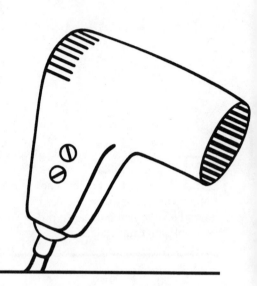

DRYING AND STYLING

As your family grows up, especially if it includes any female children, you will probably be expected to be not only the family barber, but the local stylist as well.

You may want to begin by making a part, and there's an easy way to find the natural split in your child's hair: wet it, comb it straight back, then place the palms of your hands on either side of his head and push gently forward from the back. The part will appear as if by magic.

The next step in turning a hair "cut" into a hair "style" is to dry it, and modern blow-dryers are wonderfully effective at that task. (They are also very good at blowing off stray hairs that are still clinging to a youngster's neck.) But some kids, especially very little ones, find them terrifying. Your dryer probably looks a lot like a gun—mine does—and it probably makes quite a roar at full throttle, so proceed gently and

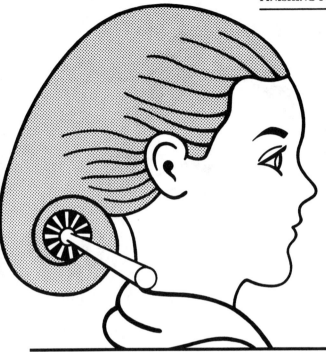

slowly. Point it at yourself first, then at a small arm or leg. If objections are raised, just let the hair dry by itself.

If the dryer is accepted—some kids think it's great fun and even tickles a little, and for them drying hair is a treat—operate it only on "low" for children, and keep it a good eight inches away from their heads. The heat generated by one of those machines is considerable and can damage both hair and skin.

The basic premise of blow-drying is to get the hair almost dry, then as a final step to introduce curls or waves. It's a technique that takes a lot of practice to master, especially on yourself. It's slightly easier when you're doing it to someone else. Do invest in a couple of round brushes, and then simply wrap the hair you want to curl around the brush and aim the dryer at it, moving the machine all the time and keeping it focused for brief stretches only.

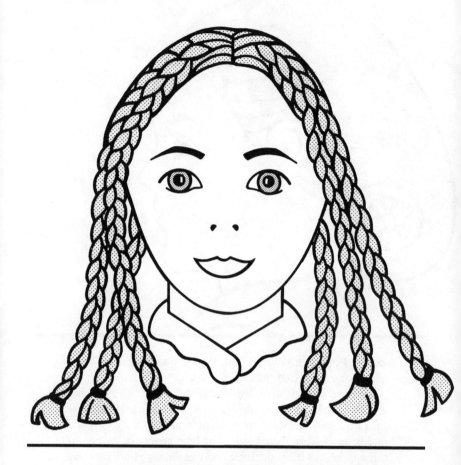

If static electricity is a problem — and it certainly can be, especially in the winter — try spraying your brush or comb with a little hair spray before you start styling.

Another way to create waves in a little girl's hair, if it's long enough, is to braid the hair while it's still damp and allow it to dry braided. A couple of fat braids will produce loose waves; a lot of thin braids will produce more pronounced curls. (Start the braids as close to the hairline as possible, of course, for the most natural-looking results.)

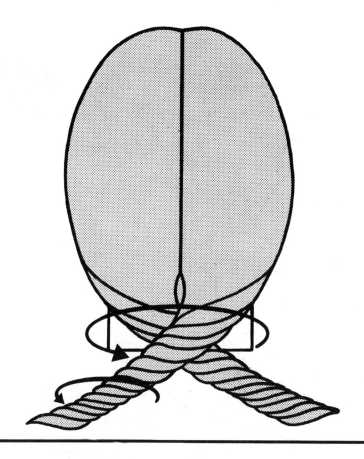

For a child who insists on long hair but who won't sit still for the time it takes to braid it in the customary fashion, you might try twist-braids.

Part the hair down the center, front to back. Twist each section round and round into a "rope" as though you were screwing in a lightbulb; then twist the "ropes" together and secure at the bottom with a coated rubber band or a strong barrette. Presto—instant neat (for at least half an hour).

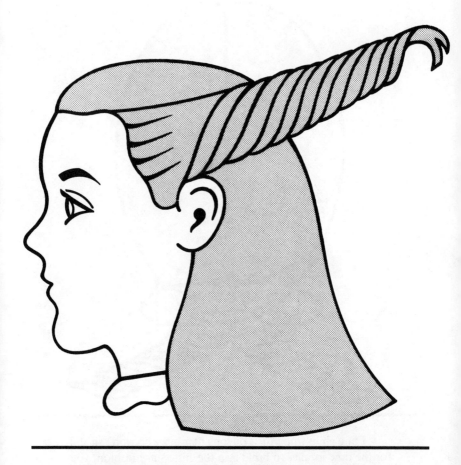

If bangs are not a part of your daughter's hairstyle and she has hair in her face from morning till night, take those two unruly sections at either side of her face, twist each one (you might braid them if you're feeling ambitious, but it's not necessary), and then secure the two of them at the crown with a barrette.

And for a party look on long hair, part it down the

center from front to back, then make one big braid above each ear (farther forward than you would if you were doing pigtails).

Pull the braids back low, along the hairline, and anchor them at the nape of the neck as securely as you can. She'll look chic and wonderful as she arrives at the party, and even

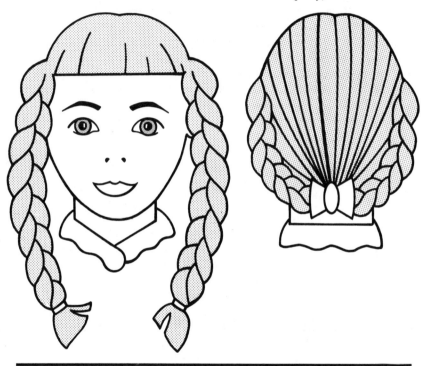

if the whole thing comes down, at least the hair is still in braids!

One final word on braids, pony tails, and little girls: although the temptation exists to do her hair up so that it *stays*, do be careful about pulling it back too tight. A lot of tension on her hair over a period of time can cause headaches and even hair loss. A little sloppiness is certainly preferable.

PERMS AND RINSES

If you've got a small daughter (not *too* small, please) who really yearns for natural curls, but who has been blessed, instead, with stick-straight hair, there is always the permanent wave. The advantages are obvious — the results are, in fact, permanent (until the hair grows out), so the daily fussing required should be drastically diminished. But take care — although the home permanent products on the market are all perfectly safe if used as directed, they do contain strong chemicals. Follow the directions, and *do* the patch test for allergies (kids are far more prone to allergic reactions than grown-ups.) Choose the degree of curl you want, and don't leave the solution on for an instant longer than indicated. A permanent imparts body to the hair, and it also dries it out — Plan to use extra conditioners and a very wide-toothed comb afterward to minimize breakage.

I would recommend permanents only for the most patient and/or motivated children, since the roll-up process is tedious and time-consuming, yet absolutely crucial for a good result. A sloppy roll-up is guaranteed to produce a frizzy perm, and what your daughter wants are *curls*, not kinks. With that in mind, read the packages carefully, and choose a product that looks easy to roll up — perhaps one with little sponges instead of little squares of slippery tissue paper. I'm told that present-day perms are virtually odorless, which is a boon. When *I* was an eight-year-old with a burning desire to be Shirley Temple, the process smelled *horrible*, and so did the whole house for days afterward.

Once you have successfully administered a permanent to your offspring, the next question may be: How do you grow it out gracefully? First of all, do regular trims, keeping up with the growth of the hair. Next, to minimize the line where the curl starts, try ribbons, headbands, and barrettes to pull the front hair back smoothly. Braiding also provides attractive camouflage, and don't overlook the obvious solution (especially if the perm was less than a roaring sucess): perhaps it's time for a nice short cut. Then you can start all over again.

Beyond permanent waves, there are not many chemical processes that I would suggest for a child's hair. For extremely curly tresses, there *are* straightening solutions, but I'm told that the chemicals involved are even stronger than perming lotions, and that they're not recommended for children. Nor are chemical tints or dyes a good idea for young hair, but there are a few tried–and–true natural color enhancers you and your daughter might like to experiment with. For blonde hair, try half and half lemon juice and water in a spray bottle, applied for ten minutes before shampooing. Or use camomile tea as an after-shampoo rinse. Cooled espresso coffee is said to provide sparkle to brunette hair; just use it as a rinse after shampooing, followed with a cool water rinse. And redheads swear by a rinse with cooled strongly brewed tea to bring out highlights.

NATURAL DISASTERS

For all manner of things that will almost certainly become stuck or entangled in your children's hair before they leave home at eighteen or thereabouts — gum, glue, a glob of paint — here's the first technique to try: hold an ice cube over the offending item until it's good and cold. See if it won't peel off at that point. If not, apply the ice for a while longer; then pour on some baby oil and slide the lump off. Finally, brush on diluted lemon juice to remove the oil and/or shampoo the head.

The bottom line with chewing gum, of course, is that you might have to cut it out — in which case, consider one of the styles in this book that's *considerably* shorter than your child's current hairdo. But there are other possibilities. An approach I haven't tried, but one that would be a hit with the kids, I suspect, is to work some peanut butter into the hair along with the gum, then comb out both substances and follow with a shampoo. Other media suggested besides peanut butter are cold cream and olive oil, depending on how you would like your child to smell.

Approach glue with the same arsenal of weapons, unless the disaster involves one of the superbond glues. They are another story altogether, and should be locked up in the medicine chest or the cleaning-supply cabinet or wherever you keep things the kids absolutely must not get into. A mess involving Crazy Glue qualifies as a medical emergency!

And then there's self-barbering. I don't think anyone gets through childhood without trying out the scissors on his own head of hair — or his baby sister's. A friend woke up in the middle of the night to discover her four-year-old standing by the bed wreathed in smiles and a very odd near-crewcut. The bad news was that the child was a little girl; the good news was that her mother woke up. The kid's stated intention was to give Mommy a trim next!

Of course, you will attempt to keep sharp scissors out of the reach of inventive youngsters, but you may still find them playing barber with the round-nose paper scissors that came with the *Sesame Street Craft Kit*. You will tell them that their enthusiasm, while commendable, is misguided, or words to that effect. And then you will assess the damage. The most common result is half a bang. Suddenly one side of your child's perfectly trimmed bangs no longer exists; it's half an inch long.

Or, if you're lucky, there are the beginnings of bangs where none were before. (You just finish the job neatly, regardless of face type.) Kids rarely attack the back of their hair, for obvious reasons: you can see the back, but they can't. They cut what they can see.

The primary approach is to try and even out the mess. Remember that the goal of any haircut is symmetry—right and left, front and back should balance each other out. Try a new cut—a shorter one, or a layered one—that will hide the damage. And finally, bear in mind the solace of anyone who's trying to learn hair cutting in the first place: hair can be depended upon to grow. In a month or two, you won't notice your child's mistakes, or your own, for that matter! Nature will have taken care of things, and you can try again.

ON PERSEVERANCE

Haircutting is not a skill you will perfect overnight. To be honest, it's something that's easier to write about than to do! But after nearly a year of practice, I think my two boys sport eminently acceptable, professional-looking heads of hair.

What remains a mystery to me is why, on one occasion, the barbering process is an enjoyable, gala event; while on the next it is suddenly viewed as a particularly devilish form of torture. I am not responsible for the volatile moods of small children—especially not my own. In fairness, there have been minor mishaps in the course of our mutual barbering adventure —I have discovered that the earlobe, when barely touched with the point of the scissors, can produce a ridiculous amount of blood. (No pain was felt, of course, until the wounded subject noticed the blood in the mirror, at which point he decided he was mortally injured.) Try to maintain grace under pressure if such misfortune should befall you, and don't feel guilty. Your child has already—or certainly will have—incurred worse damage learning to ride a two-wheeler.

As you practice and become more confident at hair-cutting, you will probably find yourself making adjustments in the styles you create. I have found, for instance, that the one-length cut works best on my boys if the sections near the crown are cut slightly longer than the front and nape-of-the-neck sections (to accomodate the family cowlick). So the cut, as I practice it, isn't quite all "one length." As is the case with cooking, I like a little leeway within the framework of a tried-and-true recipe.

But an appealing aspect of the whole hair-cutting process is that, unlike cooking, you never have a disaster so complete you have to throw it away! Time will take care of your slips, and your children will amost certainly forgive you—probably in time for the next trim.

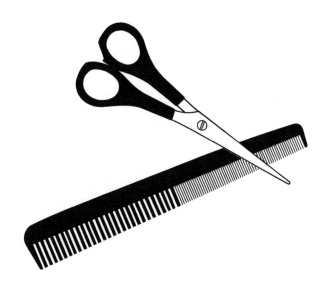